EHLERS DANLOS SYNDROME

Understanding EDS types and subtypes, causes, prevention and treatment options.

Tammy R. Brewster

TABLE OF CONTENTS

INTRODUCTION 5

CHAPTER ONE 11

What is Ehlers-Danlos Syndrome? 11

   How EDS Affects a Person 13

CHAPTER TWO 17

Types of Ehlers-Danlos Syndrome 17

CHAPTER THREE 23

Causes and Prevention of Ehlers-Danlos Syndrome 23

   Causes of Ehlers-Danlos Syndrome 23

   Prevention of Ehlers-Danlos Syndrome 25

CHAPTER FOUR 29

Life Expectancy of Ehlers-Danlos Syndrome 29

   Factors Influencing Life Expectancy 30

CHAPTER FIVE 35

Facial Features of Ehlers-Danlos Syndrome 35

   Common Facial Features 35

   Emotional and Social Impact 38

Managing Facial Features 39

CHAPTER SIX..**41**

Treatment of Ehlers-Danlos Syndrome..............................**41**

Medical Management..41

Supportive Care...44

Lifestyle Adjustments 45

CHAPTER SEVEN **47**

Exercises for Ehlers-Danlos Syndrome Patients **47**

Importance of Exercise for EDS 47

Types of Safe Exercises 48

Tips for Exercising with EDS 51

CHAPTER EIGHT **53**

Frequently Asked Questions about Ehlers-Danlos Syndrome **53**

Conclusion...**62**

INTRODUCTION

I begin by asking, "Why aren't many medical professionals familiar with Ehlers-Danlos syndrome?"

Consider this: of all the things you learn in medical school, you pay the most attention to the most common, dangerous, and actionable issues. EDS is uncommon (or was assumed to be until recently, when they began diagnosing any hypermobile person who met the Beighton Criteria for Hypermobile EDS), and they can't do much about the majority of EDS types. The majority of patients with EDS have forms for which there are no therapies available.

When John Ritter died of vascular EDS, the Ritter Rules posters were shown in ERs around the country, and I believe clinicians became more conscious of the risk of aortic dissection in someone who did not have a Marfan body type. I am not sure if they are also more aware of the risk of organ rupture.

Then there are forms of EDS that appear at birth or shortly thereafter. I'm not sure how well these are recognized by paediatricians because I've had limited experience with that side of medicine. These are rare enough; however, if a child is born with dislocated hips or any of the other odd EDS varieties, I'm sure doctors will be on whatever their version of "Google" is and investigate the unusual thing they're witnessing.

This leaves us hypermobile. Many doctors and physical therapists continue to believe that being hypermobile is a good thing, in contrast to all the stiff patients they see who are unable to perform the necessary stretches and postures to enhance their physical health. Only a few are aware of how awful some hypermobile people may get. When they come in for help, they may be unaware that a hypermobile patient requires a completely different sort of physical therapy, with small weights, low repetitions, and rigorous form to avoid joint overextension. PT is about everything that can benefit us. A doctor or therapist can administer anti-inflammatory medications, but they can do little else for hypermobile patients.

My theory is that when doctors don't have any tools to assist you, they don't learn about the disease during medical school. This is easily shown by the example of lymphedema, which is the swelling of a limb or body component caused by lymphatic malfunction. Unless you have swollen limbs as a result of cancer treatment, you may go years or decades without receiving any treatment from a doctor. Older doctors will tell you that the lymphatic system was only taught briefly in medical school. Other than specialised massage and compression, there is no treatment for it, and doctors do not perform those procedures; some may be unaware that it is available. Manual lymphatic drainage treatments are provided by specially trained occupational or physical therapists.

My sister's calves measured 57 cm (almost 22 inches) in circumference, and the doctor who visited her at the workers' compensation clinic following a fall at work kept asking me, "What's wrong with her legs?" "What do your doctors say about your legs?" "Don't your doctors do something about your legs?" No, my doctors have never asked about my legs, told her there was anything wrong with her legs, or addressed the size of her legs—except for one vascular doctor 15 years ago who prescribed her first compression stockings because he said she had venous stasis, despite the fact that she passed every doppler test she received. You believe that having normal dopplers would make a doctor question what else was going on. If he diagnosed or suspected lymphedema, he never told my sister. Given that doctors can miss legs with 22" calves, is it odd that they neglect hypermobility that cannot be seen?

Do you know who diagnosed my sister's lymphedema? A stocking-fitter. She advised her to seek a doctor's prescription to see a specialist occupational therapist at a local hospital who was Polish and had been educated in Europe to treat lymphedema. She requested that the next doctor she saw write a prescription for lymphedema treatment for her. I told that story to the doctor at the workers' compensation clinic. Two years later, when she struggled to work on her swollen legs, I utilised the internet to locate a lymphedema treatment centre three hours away, one of four in the US. I scheduled an appointment for my sister the day before Memorial Day weekend in 2015, and she was seen by a nurse practitioner.

She diagnosed her with lipedema and secondary lymphedema, which are caused by the lipedema. I assumed at the time that lipedema was just "fat in the legs," but she explained that it is fat legs out of proportion to the rest of the body, that one can be skinny elsewhere and have lipedema, and that it is not caused by overeating. Additional online research told me much more about it. I attended a national conference in 2018 and saw a speaker who was a doctor who focused on lipedema! She was the only one in the USA at the time. We have a few of them presently.

Given my sister's experiences with lipedema, lymphedema, and EDS, I've come to feel that if doctors don't have a solution (drugs, chemo, surgery), it doesn't exist in their thoughts.

CHAPTER ONE

What is Ehlers-Danlos Syndrome?

Ehlers-Danlos Syndrome (EDS) is a collection of genetic disorders that primarily affect the connective tissues in the body. Connective tissues provide support in skin, bones, blood vessels, and many other organs and tissues. They play a critical role in maintaining the structural integrity and function of various systems within the body.

EDS is characterised by a defect in the structure, production, or processing of collagen, which is a vital protein in connective tissues. Collagen acts like a glue that holds the body together, providing strength and elasticity. When collagen is faulty, the connective tissues can become fragile and stretchy, leading to a variety of medical issues.

EDS is inherited, meaning it is passed down through families. The specific genetic mutations responsible for EDS impact the way collagen is synthesised and assembled in the body. This results in the diverse range of manifestations seen in EDS patients.

The syndrome affects individuals differently, and its severity can range from mild to life-threatening. The primary focus in understanding EDS is recognizing the central role of collagen and connective tissue integrity in maintaining overall health. The disruption of these key components due to genetic mutations underpins the complexities associated with EDS.

People with Ehlers-Danlos syndrome typically have hyperflexible joints and stretchy, delicate skin. This can be a problem if you have a wound that requires stitches, as the skin is typically not tough enough to hold them.

A more severe type of the illness, known as vascular Ehlers-Danlos syndrome, can produce ruptured blood vessels, intestinal, or uterine walls. Because vascular Ehlers-Danlos syndrome can cause major problems during pregnancy, you should consult a genetic counsellor before starting a family.

In essence, Ehlers-Danlos Syndrome highlights the crucial function of connective tissues in the body and the profound impact that genetic variations can have on this intricate system.

How EDS Affects a Person

Ehlers-Danlos Syndrome (EDS) affects individuals in various ways, primarily due to its impact on connective tissues. Here are the detailed effects:

1. Joint Issues:

> Hypermobility: Joints are overly flexible and can move beyond the normal range, leading to frequent dislocations and subluxations.

> Chronic Pain: Persistent joint pain and discomfort are common due to instability and frequent injuries.

2. Skin Manifestations:

> Stretchy Skin: The skin can stretch more than usual and may feel velvety or soft.

> Fragile Skin: Skin can tear or bruise easily, and wounds may take longer to heal, often leaving scars.

3. Vascular Complications:

> ➤ Fragile Blood Vessels: Blood vessels can be more prone to rupturing, leading to serious complications such as internal bleeding.

> ➤ Easy Bruising: Individuals may bruise more easily due to fragile blood vessels and skin.

4. Musculoskeletal Problems:

> ➤ Muscle Pain and Fatigue: Constant strain on muscles to stabilise joints can lead to muscle pain and fatigue.

> ➤ Skeletal Deformities: Issues like scoliosis (curvature of the spine) and flat feet can occur.

5. Gastrointestinal Issues:

> ➤ Digestive Problems: EDS can affect the gastrointestinal tract, leading to symptoms like abdominal pain, constipation, or diarrhoea.

> ➤ Hernias: Weak connective tissues can result in hernias, where an organ pushes through an opening in the muscle or tissue that holds it in place.

6. Cardiac Concerns:

➤ Heart Valve Problems: Some types of EDS can affect heart valves, causing conditions like mitral valve prolapse.

➤ Aneurysms: There is an increased risk of aneurysms (a bulge in the wall of an artery) due to weakened blood vessel walls.

7. Dental and Oral Health:

➤ Gum Disease: Fragile gum tissue can lead to frequent gum disease.

➤ Fragile Teeth: Teeth may be more prone to cavities and other dental issues.

8. Neurological Symptoms:

➤ Nerve Compression: Joint instability and musculoskeletal issues can lead to nerve compression, causing symptoms like numbness or tingling.

➤ Headaches: Frequent headaches or migraines can occur due to joint issues in the neck and back.

9. Psychological Impact:

> ➤ Mental Health: Living with chronic pain and the physical limitations of EDS can contribute to anxiety, depression, and other mental health challenges.

> ➤ Quality of Life: The unpredictability of symptoms and the need for constant management can affect daily activities and overall quality of life.

CHAPTER TWO

Types of Ehlers-Danlos Syndrome

Ehlers-Danlos Syndrome (EDS) encompasses a group of related disorders, each with its own unique set of characteristics and challenges. Understanding the different types of EDS is crucial for proper diagnosis, management, and support. Here, let's look into the various types, highlighting not only the medical aspects but also the human experiences behind them.

Classical EDS (cEDS)

Classical EDS is marked by extremely elastic, velvety skin that can tear easily and leaves scars that resemble cigarette paper. The hypermobility of joints often leads to frequent dislocations and chronic pain. For those with cEDS, everyday activities can be a constant battle against the fear of injury and the pain that follows. Simple actions like playing with children or enjoying a walk can become daunting tasks, overshadowed by the fragility of their own bodies.

Hypermobility EDS (hEDS)

Hypermobility EDS is the most common type and is characterised by joint hypermobility, chronic pain, and a tendency for joints to dislocate easily. Individuals with hEDS often face a lifetime of persistent pain and fatigue, which can lead to feelings of frustration and helplessness. The uncertainty of when the next dislocation or injury will occur can make planning for the future feel like a fragile endeavour, filled with anxiety and the need for constant vigilance.

Vascular EDS (vEDS)

Vascular EDS is one of the most severe forms, affecting the walls of blood vessels, intestines, and uterus. People with vEDS live under the constant threat of life-threatening complications, such as arterial or organ rupture. The diagnosis of vEDS can bring a profound emotional toll, as individuals grapple with the knowledge that their condition can turn critical without warning. Every day becomes a balancing act of cherishing life's moments while managing the ever-present risk of sudden medical emergencies.

Kyphoscoliotic EDS (kEDS)

Kyphoscoliotic EDS is characterised by severe curvature of the spine (kyphoscoliosis), muscle weakness, and fragile eyes that can lead to vision problems. For those with kEDS, the physical deformities and disabilities can lead to feelings of isolation and self-consciousness. The struggle to maintain mobility and independence often requires tremendous resilience and determination, as they navigate a world not always accommodating to their needs.

Arthrochalasia EDS (aEDS)

Arthrochalasia EDS involves severe joint hypermobility and recurrent dislocations, often from birth. Individuals with aEDS face a lifetime of orthopaedic issues, including early-onset osteoarthritis. The constant cycle of joint problems and surgeries can be emotionally draining, as each step forward may feel undermined by another setback. Yet, within these challenges lies a profound strength, as individuals with aEDS continually adapt and find ways to move forward.

Dermatosparaxis EDS (dEDS)

Dermatosparaxis EDS is a rare form that leads to extremely fragile skin, severe bruising, and sagging skin. For those with dEDS, the visible signs of the condition can affect self-esteem and social interactions. The vulnerability of their skin requires meticulous care and caution, turning routine activities into potential hazards. Despite these challenges, the resilience shown by individuals with dEDS is a testament to their inner strength and determination to live life fully.

Other Rare Types

There are several other rare types of EDS, each with its own specific symptoms and challenges. These include brittle cornea syndrome (BCS), spondylodysplasia EDS (spEDS), and musculocontractural EDS (mcEDS), among others. Each type adds another layer to the complexity of EDS, and each person's experience is unique. The rarity of these conditions often means that individuals may feel isolated or misunderstood, underscoring the importance of community and support.

Living with EDS

Living with EDS means more than just managing a medical condition; it means navigating a world that often doesn't understand the silent struggles behind the visible symptoms. It's about finding strength in vulnerability, courage in adversity, and hope in the face of uncertainty. For those affected by EDS, every day is a testament to resilience and the human spirit's capacity to endure and thrive despite the odds.

CHAPTER THREE

Causes and Prevention of Ehlers-Danlos Syndrome

Understanding the causes and exploring the prevention of Ehlers-Danlos Syndrome (EDS) requires delving into the intricate world of genetics and connective tissue biology. This journey is marked by scientific complexity and the profound impact these disorders have on the lives of those affected.

Causes of Ehlers-Danlos Syndrome

Ehlers-Danlos Syndrome is primarily caused by genetic mutations that affect the production, structure, or processing of collagen and other components of connective tissue. Here's a detailed look at the underlying causes:

1. Genetic Mutations:

- ➢ EDS is usually inherited in an autosomal dominant or autosomal recessive pattern, depending on the type. In autosomal dominant inheritance, a single copy of the altered gene from one parent is sufficient to cause the disorder. In autosomal recessive inheritance, two copies of the altered gene, one from each parent, are necessary.

➢ The mutations occur in genes responsible for the synthesis and assembly of collagen, a key protein that provides strength and elasticity to connective tissues. Commonly affected genes include COL1A1, COL1A2, COL3A1, COL5A1, COL5A2, and others, depending on the specific type of EDS.

2. Collagen Defects:

➢ Collagen is a major structural protein in the body, acting as a scaffold that supports tissues and organs. Mutations in collagen genes disrupt its normal structure, leading to weakened connective tissues that are prone to stretching, tearing, and injury.

➢ Different types of collagen are affected in various forms of EDS. For instance, mutations in the COL3A1 gene lead to vascular EDS, affecting the blood vessels, skin, and internal organs.

3. Enzymatic Defects:

> ➢ Some types of EDS are caused by defects in enzymes involved in the processing of collagen. For example, kyphoscoliotic EDS (kEDS) is caused by mutations in the PLOD1 gene, which encodes an enzyme important for collagen cross-linking, essential for the stability and function of collagen fibres.

Prevention of Ehlers-Danlos Syndrome

Currently, there is no known way to prevent Ehlers-Danlos Syndrome, as it is a genetic condition. However, there are strategies to manage risks and improve quality of life for those with EDS and their families:

1. Genetic Counselling:

> ➢ Genetic counselling is crucial for families affected by EDS. It helps individuals understand the inheritance patterns, the likelihood of passing the disorder to their children, and the implications for family planning.
>
> ➢ Through genetic testing, potential parents can gain insight into their carrier status and the risk of having a

child with EDS. This information can guide informed decisions about family planning and prenatal testing options.

2. Early Diagnosis and Intervention:

- ➢ Early diagnosis is key to managing EDS effectively. Recognizing symptoms early allows for timely interventions that can prevent complications and improve outcomes.

- ➢ Regular monitoring and proactive management of symptoms can reduce the impact of EDS on daily life. This includes routine check-ups with healthcare providers familiar with EDS, physical therapy to strengthen muscles and support joints, and lifestyle modifications to minimise injury risk.

3. Education and Awareness:

- ➢ Raising awareness about EDS among healthcare professionals and the general public can lead to earlier recognition and better management of the condition. Education initiatives can help reduce the stigma and misunderstandings associated with EDS.

➢ Empowering patients with knowledge about their condition enables them to advocate for their own health and seek appropriate care.

4. Lifestyle Adjustments:

➢ Individuals with EDS can take steps to protect their joints and skin by avoiding high-impact activities, using supportive devices, and adopting ergonomic practices.

➢ Maintaining a healthy diet and staying hydrated can support overall connective tissue health. Adequate nutrition, including sufficient vitamin C, is essential for collagen production and repair.

5. Ongoing Research:

➢ Supporting and staying informed about ongoing research into EDS can provide hope for future advances in treatment and management. Research efforts are aimed at understanding the underlying mechanisms of EDS, developing targeted therapies, and potentially finding ways to correct or mitigate the genetic defects.

While EDS cannot be prevented, understanding its causes and focusing on proactive management can make a significant difference in the lives of those affected. This journey, though complex and challenging, is one of resilience and hope, guided by the advances in medical science and the strength of the human spirit.

CHAPTER FOUR

Life Expectancy of Ehlers-Danlos Syndrome

As a professional medical practitioner, it's important to address the concerns surrounding life expectancy for individuals with Ehlers-Danlos Syndrome (EDS) with clarity and compassion. EDS encompasses a diverse group of genetic disorders, each with unique challenges that can impact life expectancy in different ways.

General Considerations

For most types of EDS, life expectancy is not significantly reduced. Many individuals with EDS live full, active lives with proper management and medical care. However, the severity and specific symptoms can vary widely, and this variability influences overall health outcomes.

Factors Influencing Life Expectancy

1. Type of EDS:

- ➤ Classical EDS (cEDS) and Hypermobility EDS (hEDS): These are generally associated with a normal life expectancy. Individuals with these types can experience chronic pain, joint dislocations, and skin issues, but these symptoms, while impactful, do not typically shorten lifespan.

- ➤ Vascular EDS (vEDS): This type is the most severe and can significantly impact life expectancy. vEDS affects the blood vessels, intestines, and other organs, making them prone to spontaneous rupture. Early diagnosis and vigilant medical care are crucial for managing risks and extending life expectancy.

2. Complications:

- ➤ Cardiovascular Issues: Certain types of EDS, particularly vEDS, can lead to serious cardiovascular complications, such as arterial ruptures or dissections, which can be life-threatening if not promptly managed.

- ➤ Orthopaedic Issues: Chronic joint problems and musculoskeletal issues can lead to reduced mobility and associated health complications, but they are typically manageable with appropriate interventions.

3. Management and Medical Care:

- ➢ Early Diagnosis and Monitoring: Early and accurate diagnosis, combined with regular monitoring by specialists familiar with EDS, is key to managing the condition effectively and preventing complications.

- ➢ Proactive Treatment: Tailored treatment plans, including physical therapy, pain management, and surgical interventions when necessary, can significantly improve quality of life and overall health outcomes.

- ➢ Lifestyle Adaptations: Individuals with EDS can take proactive steps to protect their joints, skin, and overall health, such as avoiding high-impact activities, using protective gear, and maintaining a healthy lifestyle.

4. Support Systems:

- ➢ Multidisciplinary Care: Comprehensive care involving a team of healthcare professionals—such as geneticists, cardiologists, rheumatologists, orthopaedic surgeons, and physical therapists—ensures that all aspects of EDS are addressed.

➤ Community and Family Support: Emotional and social support from family, friends, and support groups can greatly enhance the quality of life and mental well-being of individuals with EDS.

Vascular EDS (vEDS)

Vascular EDS deserves special mention due to its potential impact on life expectancy. Individuals with vEDS face significant risks due to the potential for arterial, intestinal, or uterine rupture. The average life expectancy for those with vEDS is lower than for other types of EDS, often due to sudden and severe complications. However, with advancements in medical monitoring, early intervention, and lifestyle adjustments, many individuals with vEDS are living longer, healthier lives than previously anticipated.

Hope and Advances

While EDS presents many challenges, ongoing research and advancements in genetic medicine hold promise for improved treatments and outcomes. Understanding the genetic basis of

EDS and developing targeted therapies can help manage symptoms more effectively and reduce the risk of severe complications.

In essence, the life expectancy of individuals with Ehlers-Danlos Syndrome varies depending on the type and severity of the condition. With proper diagnosis, comprehensive care, and proactive management, many people with EDS can lead long and fulfilling lives. The medical community continues to strive for better understanding and treatment of EDS, offering hope for even better outcomes in the future.

CHAPTER FIVE

Facial Features of Ehlers-Danlos Syndrome

Ehlers-Danlos Syndrome (EDS) can affect various parts of the body, including the face. While the presentation of facial features can vary widely depending on the type of EDS, there are some common characteristics that may be observed. Understanding these features can help with early recognition and diagnosis, as well as provide insight into the diverse ways EDS manifests.

Common Facial Features

1. Skin Texture and Elasticity:
- Soft, Velvety Skin: Individuals with EDS often have skin that feels unusually soft and velvety. This is due to the abnormal collagen in the skin, which affects its texture.

➢ Hyperelasticity: The skin may be more stretchy than normal. This increased elasticity is often noticeable in areas like the cheeks and neck.

2. Eyes:

➢ Epicanthal Folds: Some individuals with EDS, particularly those with the classical type (cEDS), may have epicanthal folds, which are small folds of skin on the inner corners of the eyes.

➢ Prominent Eyes: Due to the lack of adequate connective tissue support, the eyes can appear more prominent or bulging.

➢ Blue Sclera: The whites of the eyes (sclera) may have a blue tint because of the thinness and transparency of the connective tissue.

3. Nose and Ears:

➢ Thin Nose: The bridge of the nose may appear thin due to the underlying connective tissue abnormalities.

➢ Thin, Translucent Skin: The skin over the nose and ears can be thin and translucent, sometimes showing underlying veins.

➢ Large or Small Ears: Ear size can vary, with some individuals having larger or smaller ears than average.

4. Mouth and Teeth:

➢ High Palate: A high, narrow palate (roof of the mouth) is common in many types of EDS, which can sometimes affect speech and dental alignment.

➢ Gum Recession: Gum tissue may be more prone to recession, leading to dental issues.

➢ Fragile Teeth: Teeth may be more prone to cavities and other dental problems due to the connective tissue abnormalities.

5. Jaw and Chin:

➢ Small Chin (Micrognathia): Some individuals with EDS may have a smaller or receding chin, which can be a noticeable facial feature.

➢ Temporomandibular Joint (TMJ) Issues: The jaw joint can be affected, leading to pain, clicking, or dislocation.

Emotional and Social Impact

The facial features associated with EDS can affect individuals in various ways beyond the physical aspects. Social interactions, self-esteem, and psychological well-being can all be influenced by how these features are perceived by others and by the individuals themselves.

- ➤ Self-Perception: Individuals with noticeable facial features of EDS may feel self-conscious or different. This can impact their confidence and social interactions.
- ➤ Social Stigma: Visible differences can sometimes lead to misunderstandings or negative reactions from others, which can be emotionally challenging.
- ➤ Acceptance and Support: It is important for individuals with EDS to receive support and understanding from family, friends, and healthcare professionals. Building a supportive community can help mitigate the emotional impact of living with noticeable facial features.

Managing Facial Features

While the facial features associated with EDS are primarily genetic and cannot be changed, there are ways to manage and mitigate some of the associated challenges:

- ➤ Regular Dental Care: Maintaining good dental hygiene and regular visits to the dentist can help manage dental issues and prevent complications.
- ➤ Skin Care: Gentle skin care routines can help manage the delicate and elastic nature of the skin. Avoiding harsh products and protecting the skin from injuries is crucial.
- ➤ Orthodontic Treatment: For those with a high palate or dental alignment issues, orthodontic treatment may be beneficial.
- ➤ Psychological Support: Counselling or therapy can be helpful for individuals struggling with self-esteem or social anxiety related to their appearance.

CHAPTER SIX

Treatment of Ehlers-Danlos Syndrome

Treating Ehlers-Danlos Syndrome (EDS) requires a comprehensive, multidisciplinary approach tailored to the specific needs of each individual. While there is no cure for EDS, effective management can significantly improve quality of life and reduce the risk of complications. Here, I will detail the various treatment strategies, emphasising both medical and supportive care, while acknowledging the emotional journey that comes with managing this complex condition.

Medical Management

1. Pain Management:

 ➢ Medications: Pain is a common and often debilitating symptom of EDS. Nonsteroidal anti-inflammatory drugs (NSAIDs), acetaminophen, and in some cases, stronger pain medications, may be prescribed.

However, long-term use of pain medication must be carefully managed to avoid dependency and side effects.

> Topical Treatments: Topical pain relievers, such as capsaicin or lidocaine creams, can provide localised relief without the systemic side effects of oral medications.

2. Joint Stability and Mobility:

> Physical Therapy: Customised physical therapy programs are essential for strengthening muscles, improving joint stability, and enhancing mobility. A skilled physical therapist can design exercises that avoid joint overstrain and promote safe movement.

> Braces and Orthotics: Supportive devices like braces, splints, and orthotic insoles can help stabilise joints and prevent dislocations. These aids provide critical support, enabling individuals to perform daily activities with less pain and risk of injury.

3. Surgical Interventions:

- ➤ Joint Surgery: In cases of severe joint damage or recurrent dislocations, surgical intervention may be necessary to repair or stabilise the joints. Surgery is generally considered a last resort and requires careful planning to minimise risks.

- ➤ Vascular Surgery: For those with vascular EDS (vEDS), vascular surgery may be needed to manage life-threatening complications like arterial ruptures. This type of surgery demands a highly skilled surgical team familiar with the fragility of connective tissues in vEDS patients.

4. Cardiovascular Care:

- ➤ Regular Monitoring: Regular cardiovascular check-ups, including imaging studies like echocardiograms and MRAs, are vital for detecting and managing potential complications in those with vEDS or other types affecting the heart and blood vessels.

- ➤ Medication: Beta-blockers or other medications may be prescribed to reduce the stress on blood vessels and lower the risk of rupture.

Supportive Care

1. Skin and Wound Care:

> Gentle Skin Care Regimens: Using mild, non-irritating skin care products can help protect the fragile skin of EDS patients. Moisturisers can prevent dryness and reduce the risk of tears.

> Wound Management: Special attention to wound care is crucial due to the skin's tendency to bruise and tear easily. Proper cleaning, use of appropriate dressings, and prompt medical attention for deep wounds are necessary to prevent infections and promote healing.

2. Nutritional Support:

> Healthy Diet: A balanced diet rich in vitamins and minerals, particularly vitamin C which is essential for collagen synthesis, can support overall connective tissue health.

> Dietary Adjustments: For those with gastrointestinal issues, dietary adjustments and working with a nutritionist can help manage symptoms like abdominal pain, constipation, and malabsorption.

3. Psychological Support:

➤ Counselling and Therapy: Living with a chronic condition like EDS can take a significant emotional toll. Psychological support through counselling or therapy can help individuals cope with anxiety, depression, and the emotional challenges of chronic pain and physical limitations.

➤ Support Groups: Connecting with others who have EDS through support groups can provide a sense of community and shared understanding. This can be a powerful source of emotional strength and practical advice.

Lifestyle Adjustments

1. Activity Modification:

➤ Low-Impact Exercise: Engaging in low-impact activities like swimming, cycling, and yoga can help maintain physical fitness without putting excessive strain on the joints.

➤ Avoiding High-Risk Activities: It's important for individuals with EDS to avoid activities that involve heavy lifting, high-impact sports, or repetitive motions that can exacerbate joint instability and pain.

2. Home and Work Environment:

➤ Ergonomic Adjustments: Making ergonomic adjustments at home and work, such as using supportive chairs, adjustable desks, and adaptive tools, can help minimise strain and prevent injury.

➤ Safe Environment: Ensuring a safe environment by removing tripping hazards, using non-slip mats, and installing grab bars in bathrooms can reduce the risk of falls and injuries.

While living with EDS poses many challenges, ongoing research offers hope for better treatments and improved quality of life. Advances in genetic research may lead to more precise diagnostic tools and potential therapies that target the underlying genetic causes of EDS.

CHAPTER SEVEN

Exercises for Ehlers-Danlos Syndrome Patients

Exercise plays a crucial role in managing Ehlers-Danlos Syndrome (EDS), helping to improve joint stability, muscle strength, and overall well-being. However, due to the unique challenges posed by EDS, exercise routines must be carefully tailored to avoid injury and accommodate individual limitations. Here, we explore a range of safe and effective exercises for EDS patients, emphasising the importance of a personalised approach and professional guidance.

Importance of Exercise for EDS

For individuals with EDS, exercise offers numerous benefits:

➤ Joint Stability: Strengthening the muscles around joints can provide additional support and reduce the risk of dislocations and subluxations.

➤ Muscle Strength: Building muscle strength helps compensate for the weakened connective tissue, enhancing overall mobility and function.

➤ Pain Management: Regular, low-impact exercise can help manage chronic pain and reduce stiffness.

➤ Improved Circulation: Exercise promotes better circulation, which can be beneficial for overall health and particularly for vascular types of EDS.

➤ Mental Health: Physical activity is known to boost mood and reduce anxiety, which is especially important for individuals dealing with chronic health issues.

Types of Safe Exercises

1. Low-Impact Aerobic Exercise:

➤ Swimming: Swimming is highly recommended for EDS patients because the buoyancy of the water supports the body and reduces stress on the joints. Activities such as water aerobics or simply swimming laps can improve cardiovascular health and muscle tone.

➢ Cycling: Stationary or upright cycling provides a low-impact cardiovascular workout that strengthens the legs without the high risk of joint strain or injury.

➢ Walking: Walking on even surfaces can be a gentle way to improve cardiovascular health. Using supportive footwear and pacing oneself to avoid fatigue is important.

2. Strength Training:

➢ Resistance Bands: Using resistance bands can help build muscle strength gently. Exercises should focus on all major muscle groups, particularly those supporting the joints. It's important to start with low resistance and gradually increase as tolerated.

➢ Bodyweight Exercises: Modified bodyweight exercises, such as wall sits, modified push-ups, and bridges, can strengthen muscles without heavy strain on the joints. Focus on controlled, slow movements to ensure stability and reduce injury risk.

3. Flexibility and Balance Exercises:

> ➢ Yoga: Gentle yoga can enhance flexibility, balance, and muscle strength. It's crucial to practise under the guidance of an instructor familiar with EDS to avoid overstretching and joint strain.

> ➢ Pilates: Pilates focuses on core strength, stability, and controlled movements. It can be particularly beneficial for improving posture and muscle tone. Like yoga, it should be practiced with caution and preferably under professional guidance.

4. Physical Therapy:

> ➢ Tailored Programs: Working with a physical therapist who has experience with EDS is invaluable. They can create a personalised exercise program that addresses individual needs, ensuring exercises are safe and effective.

> ➢ Joint Stabilisation: Physical therapists can teach specific exercises aimed at stabilising hypermobile joints, using techniques such as proprioceptive training to enhance joint awareness and control.

Tips for Exercising with EDS

1. Start Slowly: Begin with low-intensity exercises and gradually increase the duration and intensity as tolerated. Listen to your body and avoid pushing through pain.

2. Focus on Quality: Prioritise proper form and controlled movements over quantity. Incorrect form can lead to injuries, especially in hypermobile joints.

3. Warm-Up and Cool Down: Always include a gentle warm-up to prepare your muscles and joints for exercise and a cool-down period to gradually lower your heart rate and prevent stiffness.

4. Hydrate and Rest: Stay hydrated during workouts and ensure adequate rest between exercise sessions to allow your body to recover.

5. Use Supportive Gear: Wearing supportive braces or orthotics during exercise can help stabilise joints and reduce the risk of injury.

6. Monitor Symptoms: Pay attention to any signs of joint instability, excessive pain, or fatigue. Adjust the exercise routine as needed and consult with a healthcare professional if new symptoms arise.

Emotional and Community Support

Exercising with EDS can be challenging, but with the right support and resources, it can also be empowering. Joining support groups or exercise classes specifically designed for individuals with connective tissue disorders can provide motivation, encouragement, and a sense of community.

Exercise is a vital component of managing Ehlers-Danlos Syndrome. By focusing on low-impact, strength-building, and flexibility-enhancing activities, individuals with EDS can improve their physical health and quality of life. It's essential to approach exercise with caution, seek professional guidance, and listen to your body. With the right approach, exercise can become a powerful tool in the journey to living well with EDS.

CHAPTER EIGHT

Frequently Asked Questions about Ehlers-Danlos Syndrome

As a medical practitioner, I often encounter a range of questions from patients and their families about Ehlers-Danlos Syndrome (EDS). Here are some of the most frequently asked questions, along with detailed answers to help you better understand this complex condition.

1. What is Ehlers-Danlos Syndrome (EDS)?

Answer: Ehlers-Danlos Syndrome (EDS) is a group of genetic connective tissue disorders characterised by hypermobility of the joints, hyperelasticity of the skin, and tissue fragility. There are several types of EDS, each with varying symptoms and severity.

2. How is EDS diagnosed?

Answer: EDS is diagnosed through a combination of clinical evaluation, family history, and genetic testing. A medical geneticist or a specialist familiar with connective tissue disorders typically conducts the diagnosis. Diagnostic criteria include physical signs, symptoms, and, in some cases, specific genetic mutations.

3. Is there a cure for EDS?

Answer: Currently, there is no cure for EDS. The treatment aims to alleviate symptoms, prevent problems, and improve quality of life. This includes pain management, physical therapy, and ongoing monitoring for any linked health conditions.

4. Can EDS be inherited?

Answer: Yes, EDS is a genetic disorder, meaning it can be inherited. The inheritance pattern varies depending on the type of EDS. Most forms are autosomal dominant, meaning a single copy of the altered gene from one parent can cause the disorder. Some types are autosomal recessive, requiring two copies of the altered gene, one from each parent.

5. What are the common symptoms of EDS?

Answer: Common symptoms of EDS include joint hypermobility, skin that is unusually stretchy, fragile skin that bruises easily, chronic pain, and frequent joint dislocations. Symptoms vary widely depending on the type of EDS and individual differences.

6. How can I manage joint pain and instability?

Answer: Management includes physical therapy to strengthen muscles around the joints, use of braces or orthotics to provide joint support, and pain relief through medications, hot/cold therapy, and lifestyle modifications. Avoiding activities that strain the joints is also important.

7. What precautions should I take during physical activities?

Answer: Choose low-impact exercises like swimming, cycling, or walking. Avoid high-impact sports and activities that put excessive strain on the joints. Warm-up before exercising, use proper equipment, and consider working with a physical therapist to develop a safe exercise routine.

8. Are there specific dietary recommendations for EDS patients?

Answer: While there is no specific diet for EDS, maintaining a balanced diet rich in vitamins and minerals is important. Vitamin C, in particular, supports collagen production. Staying hydrated and managing any gastrointestinal issues through dietary adjustments can also be beneficial.

9. How does EDS affect dental health?

Answer: EDS can lead to fragile gums, frequent dental cavities, and issues with the jaw joint (TMJ). Regular dental check-ups, good oral hygiene, and working with a dentist familiar with EDS are important for maintaining dental health.

10. Can EDS affect the cardiovascular system?

Answer: Yes, particularly in types like vascular EDS (vEDS), where there is an increased risk of arterial, intestinal, and organ ruptures. Regular cardiovascular monitoring, avoiding heavy lifting, and managing blood pressure are crucial preventive measures.

11. What should I do if I suspect my child has EDS?

Answer: If you suspect your child has EDS, consult with a paediatrician or a geneticist. They can perform a thorough evaluation and, if necessary, genetic testing. Early diagnosis and intervention can help manage symptoms and prevent complications.

12. Is genetic counselling available for EDS?

Answer: Yes, genetic counselling is recommended for individuals with EDS and their families. It helps in understanding the inheritance patterns, risks of passing the condition to children, and provides support in family planning decisions.

13. How does EDS impact mental health?

Answer: Living with EDS can be challenging and may impact mental health, leading to anxiety, depression, or chronic stress. Psychological support, such as counselling or therapy, and joining support groups can be beneficial for emotional well-being.

14. What resources are available for EDS patients and their families?

Answer: Various resources are available, including national and international EDS organisations, online support groups, educational materials, and specialised healthcare providers. These resources provide valuable information, support, and community connections.

15. Can EDS affect the eyes?

Answer: Yes, EDS can affect the eyes in various ways, including causing myopia (nearsightedness), blue sclera (bluish tint to the whites of the eyes), and in some cases, early-onset glaucoma or retinal detachment. Regular eye exams are important for detecting and managing these issues.

16. How does EDS impact pregnancy?

Answer: Pregnancy in women with EDS requires careful monitoring due to increased risks of complications, such as preterm labour, uterine rupture (especially in vascular EDS), and joint instability. Working closely with a healthcare provider specialising in high-risk pregnancies is crucial.

17. Can children outgrow EDS?

Answer: EDS is a lifelong genetic condition, and children do not outgrow it. However, symptoms may change over time, and with appropriate management and care, many individuals learn to adapt and improve their quality of life.

18. Are there any specific medications for treating EDS?

Answer: There are no medications specifically for treating EDS itself, but various medications can help manage symptoms. These include pain relievers, anti-inflammatory drugs, and medications for gastrointestinal or cardiovascular issues. Always consult with your doctor before starting any new drug.

19. How can I protect my skin if I have EDS?

Answer: To protect fragile skin, use gentle skincare products, avoid harsh soaps and chemicals, and moisturize regularly. Wearing protective clothing and using sunscreen can also help prevent skin damage. If wounds occur, ensure proper wound care to promote healing and prevent infections.

20. What role do genetics play in EDS?

Answer: EDS is primarily caused by mutations in genes responsible for collagen production and connective tissue structure. Genetic testing can identify specific mutations, which helps in diagnosing the type of EDS and understanding its inheritance pattern.

21. Can EDS affect the gastrointestinal system?

Answer: Yes, EDS can lead to gastrointestinal issues such as irritable bowel syndrome (IBS), chronic constipation, gastroesophageal reflux disease (GERD), and hernias. Managing diet, staying hydrated, and working with a gastroenterologist can help alleviate these symptoms.

22. How does EDS impact sleep?

Answer: Chronic pain, joint instability, and other symptoms of EDS can interfere with sleep. Strategies to improve sleep include pain management, using supportive pillows and mattresses, and establishing a regular sleep routine. Consulting with a sleep specialist may also be beneficial.

23. Can individuals with EDS work and pursue careers?

Answer: Yes, many individuals with EDS can work and have successful careers. It's important to choose a job that accommodates their physical limitations and to make necessary adjustments in the workplace, such as ergonomic furniture and flexible hours, to manage symptoms effectively.

24. What research is being done to find a cure for EDS?

Answer: Research on EDS is ongoing, focusing on understanding the genetic causes, improving diagnostic methods, and developing targeted treatments. Clinical trials and studies are exploring various aspects of EDS, with the goal of finding more effective ways to manage and potentially cure the condition in the future.

Conclusion

Understanding Ehlers-Danlos Syndrome through these additional FAQs can help patients, families, and caregivers navigate the complexities of the condition. It's essential to stay informed, seek support, and work closely with healthcare providers to manage EDS effectively and improve quality of life.

We hope this book helps you find balance, and feel empowered in managing your condition. Here's to a future filled with healthy and vibrant living. Thank you for allowing us to be part of your journey, and we look forward to hearing about your successes and seeing the positive impact this book has on your life.

Wishing you health, happiness, and a lifetime of vibrant living.

Happy Healthy Living!